TYPE 2 DIABETES
FOOD LIST

The Complete Ingredient list and Food to Avoid For Type 2 Diabetes

Harley W. Norman

Copyright © 2024 by Harley W. Norman

All rights reserved

No part of this publication may be reproduced, stored in a retrieval system. or transmitted. in and form or by any means, electronic, mechanical, photocopying, recording, or otherwise, without the prior written permission of the author. The information in this eBook is true and complete to the best

of our knowledge. All recommendations are made without guarantee on the part of the author or publisher. The author and publisher disclaim any liability in connection with the use of this information.

Table of Contents

Introduction

"Are You Ready to Take Control of Your Diabetes and Live a Life Full of Energy and Vitality?"

Unveil the Secrets to Transforming Your Health with the 'Type 2 Diabetes Food List'

Imagine waking up each morning with more energy and a clear mind, knowing exactly what foods will keep your blood sugar stable throughout the day. With the "Type 2 Diabetes Food List," you can turn this vision into reality. This book is not just a guide; it's a lifeline for managing your diabetes more effectively through informed and delicious food choices. Here's how this book can change your life:

- **Reduce Medication Dependency:** Learn how to manage your diabetes naturally, potentially reducing the need for medication.

- **Enhanced Energy Levels:** Discover foods that boost your energy naturally, without the spikes and crashes.

- **Prevent Complications:** Find out how the right diet can help prevent the serious complications that often come with diabetes.

- **Personal Empowerment:** Gain the knowledge and confidence to make choices that align with your health goals.

The Story Behind the 'Type 2 Diabetes Food List'

Marie, a 52-year-old with recently diagnosed type 2 diabetes, felt overwhelmed by the dietary changes her doctor recommended. Faced with the daunting task of overhauling her diet, she worried about giving up her favorite foods and the impact on her lifestyle. That was until she discovered the "Type 2 Diabetes Food List."

Through the book, Marie learned to understand not just what foods to eat and avoid, but why some foods affected her blood sugar differently than others. Equipped with meal plans, easy recipes, and a comprehensive understanding of the glycemic index, Marie found herself excited about food again. Each page of the book was like a conversation with a knowledgeable and compassionate expert, guiding her towards better health.

As she incorporated the suggestions from the book, Marie noticed changes. Her energy levels improved, her blood sugar readings stabilized, and she even began to enjoy the creative process of cooking healthy meals. The book provided her not just with a list of foods, but with a new approach to life.

Addressing Your Concerns

You might wonder if "Type 2 Diabetes Food List" is just another diet book. It's not. We understand that changing your diet is a challenge, and this book is designed to support you every step of the way. Here's what we offer:

- **Realistic and Sustainable Advice:** No fad diets or unrealistic restrictions. Just practical, easy-to-follow guidance.

- **Flexibility:** We know everyone's body responds differently. That's why we provide options to suit various tastes and lifestyles.

- **Scientific Backing:** Every recommendation is grounded in the latest scientific research and expert advice.

- **Support Beyond Food:** While food is a huge part of managing diabetes, we also cover other lifestyle factors that can impact your health.

Embrace a life where you feel at ease with your food choices. Manage your diabetes effectively and with confidence. Let "Type 2 Diabetes Food List" guide you to a healthier, happier you. Why wait to start feeling better? Order your copy today and take the first step towards transforming your life!

Overview of Type 2 Diabetes

Type 2 diabetes is a chronic condition characterized by insulin resistance and an inability of the body to effectively use insulin, the hormone responsible for regulating blood sugar levels. Over time, this resistance can lead to consistently high blood glucose levels, which if left unmanaged, can result in a variety of health complications such as nerve damage, kidney disease, heart disease, and vision problems.

The onset of type 2 diabetes is strongly influenced by lifestyle factors, including diet, which plays a critical role in both the development and management of the disease. Optimal dietary choices can help manage blood sugar levels, reduce the risk of complications, and improve overall health and well-being. For individuals with type 2 diabetes, it is essential to focus on a balanced diet rich in nutrients, low in fat and calories, and moderate in carbohydrates. The goal is to stabilize blood sugar levels and prevent any spikes or drastic drops that can be harmful.

The Type 2 Diabetes Food List serves as a crucial tool in this dietary management. It categorizes foods based on their potential impact on blood glucose levels, providing a detailed guide on what foods to eat and what to avoid. Foods that are recommended typically have a low to moderate glycemic index (GI) and provide sustained energy without causing rapid increases in blood sugar. These include high-fiber vegetables, whole grains, lean proteins, and healthy fats, which can aid in blood sugar control and contribute to a feeling of fullness, helping manage weight—a significant factor in diabetes management.

Conversely, the food list also highlights foods that should be limited or avoided. High-glycemic foods, such as refined sugars and processed carbohydrates, can cause quick spikes in glucose levels and offer little nutritional value. Managing the intake of these foods is crucial for preventing the short-term fluctuations and long-term health issues associated with poorly controlled glucose levels.

Incorporating the principles from the Type 2 Diabetes Food List into daily life can empower individuals to make informed food choices, actively manage their diabetes, and potentially reduce their dependence on medications. Regular consultation with healthcare providers, including dietitians or nutritionists, can further tailor the food list to meet individual dietary needs, preferences, and specific health goals. This proactive approach to dietary management is instrumental in improving quality of life for those living with type 2 diabetes.

Importance of Diet in Diabetes Management

Managing type 2 diabetes effectively requires a comprehensive understanding of how various foods impact blood sugar levels. Diet plays a crucial role in controlling this condition, as the body's ability to produce and respond to insulin is impaired, leading to elevated glucose levels. By carefully selecting foods based on their glycemic index and load, individuals can maintain steadier blood glucose levels, reducing spikes that can be harmful over time.

Carbohydrates have the most immediate impact on blood sugar levels. Foods with a low to moderate glycemic index, such as whole grains, legumes, and most vegetables, release glucose slowly into the bloodstream, preventing sudden increases that can lead to hyperglycemia. On the other hand, high glycemic foods like white bread, rice, and sugary snacks cause rapid spikes in glucose levels, which are not only dangerous but can also affect overall energy levels and mood.

Fats and proteins play supportive roles in a diabetes diet. Incorporating healthy fats from sources like avocados, nuts, and olive oil can help slow the absorption of glucose into the bloodstream, promoting blood sugar stability. Proteins are essential as they provide a source of energy without directly influencing blood sugar levels, and they help in the repair and growth of tissues.

Dietary fiber is particularly important in diabetes management. High-fiber foods, such as fruits, vegetables, and whole grains, aid in digestion and slow the absorption of sugar, helping to control blood sugar levels more effectively. Additionally, fiber promotes satiety, which can help in weight management—a crucial aspect of managing diabetes, as excess body weight can exacerbate the condition.

Meal planning is another key component of diet-based diabetes management. Eating at regular intervals helps maintain blood sugar levels and prevents the lows and highs that can occur when meals are skipped or when there's too much time between meals. Portion control is equally important; even healthy foods can lead to weight gain and increased blood sugar if eaten in excess.

Hydration also plays a vital role. Water does not impact blood sugar levels and helps in the metabolism of nutrients, thus supporting overall health and facilitating the excretion of excess glucose and toxins.

Ultimately, a diet well-suited for managing type 2 diabetes is varied and balanced, focusing on nutrient-dense foods that support insulin sensitivity and reduce inflammation. By adhering to the guidelines provided in a resource like the "Type 2 Diabetes Food List," individuals can enhance their ability to manage their condition effectively, leading to a higher quality of life and reduced risk of diabetes-related complications. This approach not only helps in stabilizing blood sugar but also contributes to heart health and overall physical and mental well-being.

How to Use This Guide

To get the most out of the "Type 2 Diabetes Food List," begin by familiarizing yourself with the basic concepts of diabetes and its relationship with diet, as outlined in the early sections of the book. Understanding these fundamentals will enhance your ability to make informed choices about the foods you eat.

The guide is structured to gradually introduce you to various food categories, starting with carbohydrates, which have the most significant impact on blood sugar levels. Each category is broken down into subcategories that list recommended foods and those to avoid. Take the time to study these lists, noting which foods you already enjoy and those you might be less familiar with.

Next, explore the meal planning and recipes section. This part of the guide is designed to help you apply the knowledge you've gained by incorporating these foods into your daily meals. Try the suggested recipes that use the foods from the "to eat" lists. These recipes are tailored to be easy to prepare and nutritious, ensuring that you not only stick to a healthy diet but also enjoy your meals.

The guide also includes a section on reading food labels, which is crucial for understanding how packaged foods can fit into your diabetes diet. Pay special attention to the sections on carbohydrates, sugars, and fiber. Practice this skill the next time you shop for groceries by comparing labels of similar products to choose the best option for your health goals.

Use the food exchange lists provided to understand how different foods can substitute for each other in recipes and meal plans. This flexibility can make your diet more varied and enjoyable, preventing the monotony that often comes with strict dietary restrictions.

Regular monitoring of your blood sugar levels as you make changes to your diet is important. This will help you see the effects different foods and meals have on your glucose levels. Keep a food and blood sugar diary as recommended in the guide. Record what you eat, when you eat, and what your blood sugar levels are at different times. Over time, this record will provide valuable insights into how your body responds to certain foods, helping you to fine-tune your diet further.

Lastly, the guide encourages you to consult with healthcare professionals. Share your progress and learnings from the guide with your dietitian or doctor. They can provide personalized advice and adjustments to your diet plan based on your health status, preferences, and any medical treatments you might be receiving.

By following these steps, you can effectively use the "Type 2 Diabetes Food List" to manage your diabetes more effectively, leading to improved blood sugar control, better overall health, and a greater sense of well-being. Remember, this guide is not just about restricting certain foods but about creating a sustainable, enjoyable way of eating that supports your health goals.

Understanding Carbohydrates

Role of Carbohydrates in Blood Sugar Control

Carbohydrates play a central role in managing blood sugar levels for individuals with type 2 diabetes. They are the body's primary source of energy and have a direct impact on blood glucose levels. When carbohydrates are consumed, the digestive system breaks them down into sugars, primarily glucose, which then enters the bloodstream. The body's response to this influx of glucose is to release insulin, a hormone produced by the pancreas, which helps cells absorb glucose and use it for energy.

For those with type 2 diabetes, the body's ability to produce or respond to insulin is impaired, leading to elevated blood sugar levels if carbohydrate intake is not managed properly. Therefore, understanding and selecting the right types of carbohydrates is crucial for effective diabetes management.

Carbohydrates are found in a variety of foods, including fruits, vegetables, grains, and dairy products. They are categorized into two groups: simple and complex. Simple carbohydrates, also known as sugars, are quickly digested and can lead to rapid spikes in blood sugar levels. These are found in foods such as soft drinks, desserts, and candy, as well as in some natural sources like fruit. While fruits contain essential nutrients and should not be entirely avoided, portion control and timing are key to managing their impact on blood sugar levels.

Complex carbohydrates, on the other hand, are found in whole grains, legumes, and starchy vegetables. These carbohydrates are made up of longer chains of sugar molecules, which take more time for the body to break down and digest. As a result, they provide a slower, more sustained release of glucose into the bloodstream, which helps maintain more stable blood sugar levels. Additionally, complex carbohydrates are typically high in fiber, which can further slow the absorption of sugar and help improve blood sugar control.

Fiber, a type of carbohydrate that the body cannot digest, plays a significant role in blood sugar control. High-fiber foods not only slow the absorption of sugar but also help to reduce cholesterol levels and promote a healthy digestive system. Incorporating a good balance of soluble and insoluble fiber from various sources can aid in managing diabetes effectively.

For effective dietary management of type 2 diabetes, carbohydrate counting is a helpful technique. It involves keeping track of the amount of carbohydrates consumed at each meal to maintain blood sugar levels within target ranges. Another useful method is understanding the glycemic index (GI) of foods. The GI measures how quickly food increases blood glucose levels; foods with a low GI value are preferable for diabetes management as they cause a slower rise in blood glucose levels.

Meal planning for diabetes should emphasize complex carbohydrates with a low to medium GI, balanced with appropriate portions of protein and healthy fats to further mitigate rapid spikes in blood sugar. By making informed choices about the types of carbohydrates consumed, individuals with type 2 diabetes can significantly improve their blood sugar control and overall health.

Different Types of Carbohydrates

Carbohydrates are a critical focus in the management of type 2 diabetes because they have the most direct impact on blood glucose levels. There are several types of carbohydrates, and understanding these can help you make informed decisions about your diet.

Simple carbohydrates are also known as sugars. These are quickly digested and absorbed, leading to rapid increases in blood sugar. Simple carbohydrates can be found naturally in foods such as fruits, milk, and milk products. They are also found in processed and refined sugars such as candy, table sugar, syrups, and soft drinks. For a diabetes-friendly diet, it's generally advised to limit these types of sugars unless they are found naturally in whole fruits and dairy, as these also provide essential nutrients and fiber which can help mitigate blood sugar spikes.

Complex carbohydrates take longer to digest and generally have a less immediate impact on blood glucose. They are found in foods such as whole grains, legumes, potatoes, and other starchy vegetables. Complex carbohydrates are beneficial because they provide a steady source of energy and have higher nutritional values, including fiber. Fiber is especially important as it can help to slow the absorption of sugar, improving blood glucose levels and aiding in digestive health.

Dietary fiber is a unique type of carbohydrate because it is not digested by the body. It is categorized into soluble and insoluble fiber. Soluble fiber dissolves in water to form a gel-like substance that can help lower blood glucose levels and reduce cholesterol. Good sources include oats, peas, beans, apples, citrus fruits, carrots, barley, and psyllium. Insoluble fiber does not dissolve in water and helps to move material through the digestive system, aiding in regular bowel movements. Sources of insoluble fiber include whole wheat flour, wheat bran, nuts, beans, vegetables, and potatoes.

Resistant starch is another form of carbohydrate that functions similarly to fiber. It resists digestion in the small intestine and ferments in the large intestine, acting as a prebiotic to feed beneficial gut bacteria. This type of starch can be found in foods like unripe bananas, cooked and cooled potatoes or rice, and legumes. It can be beneficial for blood sugar management as it does not cause sharp spikes in glucose levels.

For people with type 2 diabetes, focusing on complex carbohydrates and high-fiber foods can be particularly beneficial. These foods not only help in maintaining more stable blood glucose levels but also contribute to overall health by providing vitamins, minerals, and antioxidants.

When planning your meals, aim to include a variety of carbohydrate sources, paying particular attention to those that are less processed. Balance carbohydrate intake with healthy proteins and fats to further stabilize blood sugar levels and maintain satiety. This approach not only helps in managing day-to-day blood sugar levels but also supports long-term health goals and disease management.

Carbohydrate Counting and Glycemic Index

Carbohydrate counting is a vital tool for managing blood sugar levels and is particularly beneficial for individuals with type 2 diabetes. This method involves tracking the grams of carbohydrates consumed at each meal to manage blood glucose levels effectively. To use carbohydrate counting, it's important to first know which foods contain carbohydrates. These typically include breads, grains, fruits, vegetables, dairy products, and sweets. Once familiar with these sources, you can begin to track the total carbohydrates you eat or drink. Many people with type 2 diabetes aim to consume a consistent amount of carbohydrates at each meal, which can help in maintaining a steady blood sugar level.

The glycemic index (GI) complements carbohydrate counting by rating how quickly foods with carbohydrates raise blood sugar levels after eating. Foods are scored on a scale from 0 to 100. Foods with a high GI (greater than 70) are digested rapidly, causing a quicker and higher rise in blood sugar levels. Examples include white bread, short-grain white rice, and pastries. Medium GI foods score between 56 and 69, and low GI foods score 55 or less; these are digested more slowly, leading to a gradual rise in blood sugar. Foods like whole oats, lentils, and most fruits fall into these categories.

Combining carbohydrate counting with an understanding of the glycemic index allows for more precise management of diet and blood sugar levels. For instance, if one opts for a high-carb food, choosing one with a lower GI can mitigate some of the potential spikes in blood glucose levels. This approach not only helps in maintaining energy throughout the day but also aids in long-term management of blood glucose levels, potentially reducing the risk of diabetes-related complications.

Additionally, the concept of glycemic load (GL) can further refine dietary choices. Glycemic load considers both the glycemic index and the carbohydrate content in a serving of food to estimate how much the food will raise a person's blood glucose level after eating it. This measure can provide a more accurate representation of how foods will affect blood sugar levels. For example, watermelon has a high GI but a low GL, meaning it has less impact on blood sugar levels due to its low carbohydrate content per serving.

Understanding and implementing these concepts requires practice and awareness, but they offer a powerful means of controlling glucose levels through diet. This is especially helpful when creating meal plans or making food choices on the go, ensuring that individuals with type 2 diabetes can enjoy a wide variety of foods while still managing their condition effectively. Regular consultation with a healthcare provider or a registered dietitian can also aid in refining these practices to tailor them to individual health needs and goals.

Foods to Include

Whole Grains

Whole Grain	Nutritional Benefits	Serving Size	Cooking Time	Instructions
Quinoa	High in protein and fiber, complete amino acid profile	1/2 cup cooked	15-20 minutes	Rinse thoroughly, then simmer in water until grains are translucent and the germ has spiraled out.
Brown Rice	Rich in magnesium, phosphorus, and fiber	1/2 cup cooked	45 minutes	Rinse well and cook in water using a 2:1 ratio, simmer until tender.
Barley	High in beta-glucan fiber, can help reduce cholesterol	1/2 cup cooked	30-40 minutes	Cook in water using a 3:1 ratio until grains are tender but

Whole Grain	Nutritional Benefits	Serving Size	Cooking Time	Instructions
				chewy.
Buckwheat	Good source of antioxidants and magnesium	1/2 cup cooked	15-20 minutes	Boil water, add buckwheat, reduce to a simmer, cover, and cook until tender.
Millet	Alkaline grain, easy to digest, and high in antioxidants	1/2 cup cooked	20-25 minutes	Toast grains in a dry pan first, then add water using a 2:1 ratio and simmer until water is absorbed.
Bulgur Wheat	High in fiber and protein, quicker cooking than other whole grains	1/2 cup cooked	10-15 minutes	Boil water, add bulgur, remove from heat, cover, and let it sit until water is absorbed and grains are soft.

Whole Grain	Nutritional Benefits	Serving Size	Cooking Time	Instructions
Amaranth	Rich in protein, containing lysine, and good source of iron and calcium	1/2 cup cooked	20-25 minutes	Rinse and simmer in water using a 2:1 ratio until grains are fluffy and water is absorbed.
Oat Groats	Provides cardiovascular benefits from beta-glucan fiber	1/2 cup cooked	50-60 minutes	Simmer in water using a 4:1 ratio until tender.
Spelt	High in soluble fiber, aids in blood sugar control	1/2 cup cooked	40-60 minutes	Cook in water using a 3:1 ratio, simmer until grains are tender.
Teff	High in calcium, iron, and protein	1/2 cup cooked	15-20 minutes	Cook in water using a 3:1 ratio, simmer until it has a creamy texture.
Rye	Good source of	1/2 cup	50-60	Cook in water

Whole Grain	Nutritional Benefits	Serving Size	Cooking Time	Instructions
	soluble fiber, beneficial for weight and blood sugar management	cooked	minutes	using a 4:1 ratio, simmer until tender.
Sorghum	Gluten-free, high in antioxidants and phytochemicals that support cardiovascular health	1/2 cup cooked	50-60 minutes	Boil in water until tender. Can also be popped like popcorn.
Wild Rice	Rich in antioxidants, protein, and dietary fiber	1/2 cup cooked	45-55 minutes	Rinse thoroughly, then cook in water using a 3:1 ratio, simmer until tender.
Farro	Contains cyanogenic glucosides that help boost the immune system	1/2 cup cooked	25-30 minutes	Soak overnight, then simmer in fresh water until tender but still chewy.

Whole Grain	Nutritional Benefits	Serving Size	Cooking Time	Instructions
Kamut	High in selenium, zinc, and magnesium	1/2 cup cooked	40-60 minutes	Soak overnight, rinse, and then cook in fresh water using a 3:1 ratio until grains are tender.
Freekeh	High in protein and fiber, has a low glycemic index which is beneficial for blood sugar management	1/2 cup cooked	20-25 minutes	Simmer in water until it reaches a chewy texture.
Black Rice	High in anthocyanin antioxidants, which have potential health benefits including improving insulin sensitivity	1/2 cup cooked	30-35 minutes	Rinse well and cook in water using a 2:1 ratio, simmer until tender.

Whole Grain	Nutritional Benefits	Serving Size	Cooking Time	Instructions
Fonio	Good source of iron, protein, and fiber, fast cooking	1/2 cup cooked	5 minutes	Rinse and simmer in water using a 2:1 ratio for about 5 minutes.
Emmer Wheat	Rich in fiber, protein, and antioxidants, aids in digestion and has a low GI	1/2 cup cooked	30 minutes	Simmer in water until grains are tender and chewy.
Tritordeum	High in lutein, dietary fiber, and protein	1/2 cup cooked	30 minutes	Cook in boiling water until tender, similar to wheat berries.

This comprehensive guide to whole grains offers a variety of options that can fit into a balanced diet for managing type 2 diabetes. Each grain listed provides unique nutritional benefits and can be a part of a healthful eating plan aimed at stabilizing blood sugar and enhancing overall health.

Vegetables

Vegetable	Nutritional Benefits	Serving Size	Preparation Instructions	Cooking Time
Broccoli	High in fiber, vitamin C, and chromium	1 cup, chopped	Steam until bright green and tender	5-7 minutes
Spinach	Rich in iron, calcium, and antioxidants	1 cup, raw	Can be eaten raw or lightly steamed	2-3 minutes
Kale	High in vitamins A, C, K, fiber, and calcium	1 cup, chopped	Sauté with olive oil and garlic	5-7 minutes
Carrots	Good source of beta-carotene and fiber	1 medium carrot	Steam or eat raw for maximum benefits	8-10 minutes
Cauliflower	Low in carbs, high in fiber and B vitamins	1 cup, chopped	Roast with herbs and a sprinkle of olive oil	20-25 minutes

Vegetable	Nutritional Benefits	Serving Size	Preparation Instructions	Cooking Time
Brussels Sprouts	Rich in vitamins C and K, fiber, and folate	1 cup, halved	Roast until caramelized or steam	20-25 minutes roast, 6-8 minutes steam
Bell Peppers	High in vitamin C and antioxidants	1 cup, sliced	Stir-fry or eat raw in salads	5-7 minutes
Zucchini	Low calorie, high in potassium and manganese	1 cup, sliced	Sauté or add to stir-fries	5-7 minutes
Cucumber	Hydrating, with vitamin K and magnesium	½ cup, sliced	Serve raw or pickled	0 minutes
Tomato	Contains lycopene, vitamins C and K	1 medium tomato	Eat raw or add to salads	0 minutes
Green Beans	Good source of fiber,	1 cup	Steam or sauté with almonds	5-7 minutes

Vegetable	Nutritional Benefits	Serving Size	Preparation Instructions	Cooking Time
	vitamins A, C, and K			
Asparagus	High in folate and vitamins A, C, and K	1 cup	Grill or roast with a drizzle of olive oil	10-12 minutes
Eggplant	High in fiber and manganese	1 cup, cubed	Bake or grill with a brush of olive oil	20-25 minutes
Radishes	Low in carbs, good for hydration	1 cup, sliced	Best served raw for crunch	0 minutes
Beets	High in fiber, folate, and manganese	1 cup, sliced	Roast to bring out natural sweetness	30-40 minutes
Sweet Potatoes	Rich in beta-carotene and fiber	1 medium potato	Bake or mash	45-50 minutes bake
Swiss Chard	Excellent source of magnesium and iron	1 cup, chopped	Sauté with a touch of lemon	3-5 minutes

Vegetable	Nutritional Benefits	Serving Size	Preparation Instructions	Cooking Time
Onions	Good for heart health and anti-inflammatory	1 cup, sliced	Caramelize or add to dishes for flavor	10-15 minutes
Mushrooms	Low in carbs, good source of selenium	1 cup, sliced	Sauté with herbs and a bit of butter	8-10 minutes
Pumpkin	Rich in vitamins A and C, and fiber	1 cup, cubed	Roast or make into a soup	25-30 minutes roast

This table should serve as a practical guide for integrating a variety of vegetables into a diabetes-friendly diet, helping to manage blood sugar levels while providing necessary nutrients and enhancing meal diversity. Each vegetable listed can be prepared in ways that maintain or enhance their natural flavors and health benefits, making them a delicious and nutritious part of daily eating.

Fruits

Fruit	Serving Size	Nutritional Information (per serving)	Benefits	Notes
1. Apples	1 small apple	Approx. 77 calories, 21g carbs, 4g fiber	Low in calories, high in fiber	Eat with skin for maximum fiber
2. Pears	1 small pear	Approx. 86 calories, 23g carbs, 5g fiber	Good source of vitamin C and fiber	Ideal for snacking or adding to salads
3. Berries	1/2 cup	Approx. 32-50 calories, 11-18g carbs, 2-4g fiber	Antioxidant-rich, low in calories	Include blueberries, strawberries, and raspberries
4. Cherries	1/2 cup	Approx. 52 calories, 12.5g carbs, 1.5g fiber	Lower glycemic index	Great for snacking or in desserts
5. Peaches	1 small peach	Approx. 58 calories, 14g calories,	Rich in vitamins A	Perfect for smoothies or

Fruit	Serving Size	Nutritional Information (per serving)	Benefits	Notes
		carbs, 2g fiber	and C	salads
6. Plums	1 medium plum	Approx. 30 calories, 8g carbs, 1g fiber	Low calories	Can be eaten in fresh or stewed
7. Oranges	1 small orange	Approx. 45 calories, 11g carbs, 2g fiber	High in vitamin C	Avoid juicing to retain fiber
8. Kiwi	1 medium kiwi	Approx. 42 calories, 10g carbs, 2g fiber	High in vitamin C and E	Can be added to yogurt or salads
9. Grapefruit	1/2 medium	Approx. 52 calories, 13g carbs, 2g fiber	Helps improve insulin sensitivity	Can interact with certain medications
10. Pomegranate	1/2 cup seeds	Approx. 72 calories, 16g carbs, 3.5g fiber	Antioxidant-rich	Can be added to salads or eaten raw
11. Cantaloupe	1 cup diced	Approx. 53 calories, 13g carbs	High in vitamin A	Refreshing in a fruit salad or

Fruit	Serving Size	Nutritional Information (per serving)		Benefits		Notes	
		carbs, fiber	1.4g			on its own	
12. Apricots	3 small apricots	Approx. 51 calories, carbs, 2g fiber	12g	High potassium	in	Best consumed when fresh	
13. Bananas	1 small banana	Approx. 90 calories, carbs, fiber	23g 2.6g	High potassium and vitamin B6	in	Choose slightly green for lower GI	
14. Mangoes	1/2 cup sliced	Approx. 54 calories, carbs, fiber	14g 1.5g	High vitamin A and C	in	Ideal for tropical smoothies	
15. Grapes	1/2 cup	Approx. 52 calories, carbs, fiber	14g 0.8g	Contains resveratrol		Can be frozen for a cool snack	
16. Watermelon	1 cup diced	Approx. 46 calories, carbs,	12g 0.6g	Hydrating, low calories		Best consumed in moderation	in

Fruit	Serving Size	Nutritional Information (per serving)	Benefits	Notes
		fiber		due to high GI
17. Papaya	1 cup cubes	Approx. 55 calories, 14g carbs, 2.5g fiber	Digestive enzyme papain	Great in tropical salads or blended in smoothies
18. Pineapple	1/2 cup chunks	Approx. 40 calories, 10g carbs, 1g fiber	Rich in bromelain	Ideal for grilling or adding to fruit salads
19. Figs	2 medium figs	Approx. 74 calories, 19g carbs, 3g fiber	High in fiber	Delicious fresh or dried
20. Blackberries	1/2 cup	Approx. 31 calories, 7g carbs, 4g fiber	High in vitamins C and K	Excellent for adding to oatmeal or yogurt

Each fruit listed provides a unique blend of nutrients that can aid in managing type 2 diabetes when incorporated as part of a balanced diet. Remember to consider the overall carbohydrate content of your daily diet and adjust portions accordingly to maintain stable blood glucose levels. Eating fruits whole rather than juiced or blended is generally recommended to maximize fiber intake and reduce glycemic response.

Proteins

Protein Ingredient	Instructions	Nutritional Information	Serving Size	Cooking Time
Chicken breast	Grill or bake with herbs and spices	165 calories, 31g protein, 3.6g fat	1 medium breast	20-25 min
Turkey breast	Roast with olive oil and rosemary	153 calories, 34g protein, 0.7g fat	4 ounces	30-40 min
Salmon	Bake with lemon and dill	233 calories, 25g protein, 15g fat	4 ounces	15-20 min
Tuna (canned in water)	Mix with low-fat mayo for sandwiches	99 calories, 22g protein, 0.8g fat	4 ounces	None
Lean beef (top sirloin)	Grill or broil with a rub of spices	206 calories, 26g protein, 10g fat	4 ounces	6-8 min per side
Pork loin	Roast with garlic and thyme	190 calories, 28g protein, 8g fat	4 ounces	45-60 min

Protein Ingredient	Instructions	Nutritional Information	Serving Size	Cooking Time
Eggs	Scramble with spinach and mushrooms	72 calories, 6g protein, 5g fat (per egg)	2 eggs	5-7 min
Lentils	Boil and add to salads or soups	116 calories, 9g protein, 0.4g fat	1/2 cup cooked	15-20 min
Chickpeas	Roast with paprika and olive oil for a snack	143 calories, 6g protein, 1.3g fat	1/2 cup cooked	20-30 min roasted
Tofu	Stir-fry with vegetables in low-sodium soy sauce	86 calories, 10g protein, 5g fat	1/2 cup	5-10 min
Black beans	Simmer in chili or blend into dips	114 calories, 8g protein, 0.5g fat	1/2 cup cooked	1-2 hours simmer
Quinoa	Cook and use as a base for stir-fries	111 calories, 4g protein, 1.8g fat	1/2 cup cooked	15 min

Protein Ingredient	Instructions	Nutritional Information	Serving Size	Cooking Time
Almonds	Toast lightly and use as a salad topping	163 calories, 6g protein, 14g fat	1 ounce	5-10 min toasted
Greek yogurt (non-fat)	Serve with berries or mix into smoothies	59 calories, 10g protein, 0.4g fat	1/2 cup	None
Cottage cheese (low-fat)	Pair with fruit or use in pancakes	81 calories, 14g protein, 1g fat	1/2 cup	None
Edamame	Steam and sprinkle with sea salt as a snack	120 calories, 11g protein, 5g fat	1/2 cup shelled	5-10 min steamed
Tempeh	Marinate and bake for a meat substitute	160 calories, 15g protein, 9g fat	4 ounces	20-30 min
Sardines (canned in water)	Serve on whole-grain toast or in	191 calories, 23g protein, 10g fat	1 can (3.75 oz)	None

Protein Ingredient	Instructions	Nutritional Information	Serving Size	Cooking Time
	salads			
Skim milk	Use in oatmeal or coffee	83 calories, 8g protein, 0.2g fat	1 cup	None
Pea protein powder	Blend into smoothies or stir into oatmeal	120 calories, 24g protein, 2g fat (varies by brand)	2 tablespoons	None

This table provides a wide range of protein choices suitable for managing type 2 diabetes, allowing for diverse and flexible meal planning that can be adjusted according to personal preferences and dietary goals. Each item offers specific preparation methods, making it easy to incorporate these proteins into daily meals.

Dairy and Dairy Alternatives

Ingredient	Type	Nutritional Information (per serving)	Serving Size	Cooking Time
1. Greek Yogurt	Dairy	High in protein, low in sugar, contains probiotics	1 cup	None
2. Cottage Cheese	Dairy	Rich in protein, low in carbohydrates	1/2 cup	None
3. Skim Milk	Dairy	Low in fat, good source of vitamin D and calcium	1 cup	None
4. Almond Milk (unsweetened)	Dairy Alternative	Low in calories and carbohydrates, contains vitamin E	1 cup	None
5. Soy Milk (unsweetened)	Dairy Alternative	High in protein, contains	1 cup	None

Ingredient	Type	Nutritional Information (per serving)	Serving Size	Cooking Time
		isoflavones, vitamin D, and calcium		
6. Cheddar Cheese	Dairy	High in protein and calcium, but also in saturated fat	1 oz	None
7. Ricotta Cheese	Dairy	Low in fat, high in protein, good for spreads and fillings	1/4 cup	None
8. Mozzarella Cheese	Dairy	High in protein, calcium-rich, lower in sodium than other cheeses	1 oz	None
9. Oat Milk (unsweetened)	Dairy Alternative	Low in fat, good source of vitamin B12, often fortified	1 cup	None

Ingredient	Type	Nutritional Information (per serving)	Serving Size	Cooking Time
		with calcium		
10. Coconut Milk (unsweetened)	Dairy Alternative	High in MCTs, low in carbohydrates	1 cup	None
11. Cashew Milk (unsweetened)	Dairy Alternative	Low in calories and fat, contains magnesium	1 cup	None
12. Flaxseed Milk (unsweetened)	Dairy Alternative	High in omega-3 fatty acids, low in calories	1 cup	None
13. Hemp Milk (unsweetened)	Dairy Alternative	Contains omega-3 and omega-6 fatty acids, protein-rich	1 cup	None
14. Kefir	Dairy	Probiotic-rich, good for gut health, high in protein	1 cup	None

Ingredient	Type	Nutritional Information (per serving)	Serving Size	Cooking Time
15. Parmesan Cheese	Dairy	Low in lactose, high in calcium and protein	1 oz	None
16. Goat Cheese	Dairy	Easier to digest, lower in lactose than cow's milk cheeses	1 oz	None
17. Swiss Cheese	Dairy	High in protein and calcium, lower in sodium	1 oz	None
18. Provolone Cheese	Dairy	Good source of calcium and protein	1 oz	None
19. Gouda Cheese	Dairy	Rich in vitamins K2 and B12, high in calcium	1 oz	None
20. Lactose-Free Milk	Dairy	Provides the same nutrients as regular milk without lactose	1 cup	None

This table provides an array of options for those managing type 2 diabetes, offering both traditional dairy products and plant-based alternatives that cater to different dietary needs and preferences. Each product is chosen based on its nutritional profile, which is crucial for maintaining balanced blood sugar levels. For cooking and usage, most of these ingredients can be used directly or incorporated into various recipes, making them versatile components of a diabetic-friendly diet.

Fats

For managing type 2 diabetes effectively, incorporating healthy fats into your diet is crucial as they can help improve blood sugar control, reduce bad cholesterol levels, and enhance overall heart health.

Fat Ingredient	Nutritional Information (per serving)	Serving Size	Cooking Instructions/Tips	Cooking Time
Avocado	240 calories, 22g fat, 3g saturated fat	1 whole	Mash for spreads or slice for salads.	No cook
Almonds	164 calories, 14g fat, 1g saturated fat	1 oz (23 nuts)	Toast lightly to enhance flavor in dishes.	5-10 minutes
Olive oil	119 calories, 13.5g fat, 1.9g saturated fat	1 tbsp	Use for dressings or low-heat cooking.	No cook or varies
Walnuts	185 calories, 18.5g fat, 1.7g saturated fat	1 oz (14 halves)	Chop and add to oatmeal or yogurt.	No cook
Flaxseeds	55 calories, 4.3g fat, 0.4g	1 tbsp ground	Sprinkle ground seeds over cereal or	No cook

Fat Ingredient	Nutritional Information (per serving)	Serving Size	Cooking Instructions/Tips	Cooking Time
	saturated fat		blend into smoothies.	
Chia seeds	137 calories, 8.7g fat, 0.9g saturated fat	1 oz	Soak in water to form a gel for desserts or drinks.	No cook
Coconut oil	121 calories, 13.5g fat, 11.7g saturated fat	1 tbsp	Use for baking or stir-frying at medium heat.	Varies
Sunflower seeds	164 calories, 14g fat, 1.5g saturated fat	1 oz	Add to salads or homemade granola.	No cook
Peanut butter (natural)	188 calories, 16g fat, 3.4g saturated fat	2 tbsp	Spread on whole-grain toast or stir into oatmeal.	No cook
Sesame oil	120 calories, 13.6g fat, 1.9g saturated fat	1 tbsp	Ideal for flavoring dishes or dressings.	No cook or varies
Canola oil	124 calories, 14g fat, 1g	1 tbsp	Suitable for frying, baking, and sautéing.	Varies

Fat Ingredient	Nutritional Information (per serving)	Serving Size	Cooking Instructions/Tips	Cooking Time
	saturated fat			
Pecans	196 calories, 20.4g fat, 1.8g saturated fat	1 oz (19 halves)	Toast and add to salads or desserts.	5-10 minutes
Cashews	155 calories, 12g fat, 2.2g saturated fat	1 oz	Use in stir-fries or as a creamy base for vegan sauces.	Varies
Macadamia nuts	204 calories, 21.5g fat, 3.4g saturated fat	1 oz (12 nuts)	Blend into homemade nut butter or desserts.	No cook
Pistachios	159 calories, 12.9g fat, 1.6g saturated fat	1 oz (49 nuts)	Chop and sprinkle on baked goods or salads.	No cook
Hazelnuts	178 calories, 17g fat, 1.3g saturated fat	1 oz (21 nuts)	Roast and add to chocolates or pastries.	10-15 minutes
Pumpkin seeds	158 calories, 13.9g fat, 2.4g saturated fat	1 oz	Roast with spices for a snack or garnish.	10-15 minutes

Fat Ingredient	Nutritional Information (per serving)	Serving Size	Cooking Instructions/Tips	Cooking Time
Ghee (clarified butter)	112 calories, 12.7g fat, 8g saturated fat	1 tbsp	Use for cooking at high temperatures.	Varies
Hemp seeds	166 calories, 14.6g fat, 1.5g saturated fat	2 tbsp	Sprinkle over salads or blend into smoothies.	No cook
Grapeseed oil	120 calories, 14g fat, 1.3g saturated fat	1 tbsp	Use for dressings or high-heat cooking like stir-frying.	Varies

Each of these fats offers unique benefits and can be incorporated into various recipes to enrich flavor and boost nutritional value. Keep serving sizes in mind to maintain appropriate portion control. These healthy fats are crucial in a balanced diet for managing type 2 diabetes, contributing not only to improved blood sugar levels but also to overall heart health.

Foods to Avoid or Limit

High Glycemic Index Foods

Managing type 2 diabetes effectively includes understanding which foods to limit or avoid, particularly those with a high glycemic index (GI). High GI foods can cause rapid spikes in blood sugar levels, which can be detrimental for diabetes control.

Food	Glycemic Index (Approximate)	Reason to Avoid
White bread	70-90	Rapidly increases blood sugar due to high starch and low fiber content.
Rice cakes	82	Cause quick spikes in blood sugar due to being highly processed and lacking fiber.
Pretzels	83	High GI and often high in sodium, offering little nutritional benefit.
Corn flakes	81	Highly processed with little fiber and protein, leading to

Food	Glycemic Index (Approximate)	Reason to Avoid
		quick digestion and blood sugar spikes.
Baked potatoes	85	High starch content that leads to rapid increase in blood sugar levels.
Watermelon	72	High GI, although it has a low glycemic load, large servings can still spike blood sugar.
Pineapple	66	Quickly raises blood sugar due to its high natural sugar content and rapid digestibility.
Instant oatmeal	70	Processed to cook quickly, losing much of its natural fiber and causing quicker blood sugar increases.
Popcorn	65	Can quickly raise blood sugar if eaten in large quantities due to being a high GI snack.
Soft drinks	59-68	Contain high levels of sugar, leading to immediate and significant blood sugar spikes.

Food	Glycemic Index (Approximate)	Reason to Avoid
Fruit juices	40-66	Often contain as much sugar as soft drinks, rapidly increasing blood sugar levels.
White pasta	45-65	Refined carbs with low fiber content, leading to faster glucose absorption and blood sugar spikes.
White rice	73	Rapidly digested with little fiber, causing significant blood sugar fluctuations.
Sweetened breakfast cereals	70-85	High in sugar and often low in fiber, leading to quick blood sugar spikes.
Candy bars	70-80	High in sugar and fats, causing rapid blood sugar increases and contributing to weight gain.
Cookies and pastries	70-80	Contain refined sugars and fats, which lead to fast increases in blood sugar.
Sugary desserts	65-80	High in sugar and often fat, which can exacerbate blood

Food	Glycemic Index (Approximate)	Reason to Avoid
		glucose management issues.
French fries	75	High GI due to being deep-fried and high in simple carbohydrates.
Energy drinks	70	High sugar content that can cause quick spikes in blood sugar levels.
Honey	58-60	Although natural, it's high in simple sugars that rapidly affect blood sugar levels.

In addition to high GI foods, other foods to avoid are those high in saturated and trans fats, excessive sodium, and added sugars as they can contribute to heart disease, hypertension, and overall poor health, complicating diabetes management. By focusing on low to medium GI foods, rich in fiber, and balanced in macros, individuals with type 2 diabetes can better manage their blood sugar levels and reduce the risk of diabetes-related complications.

Processed Grains and Sugary Foods

For individuals managing type 2 diabetes, it is crucial to limit intake of processed grains and sugary foods. These items can cause rapid spikes in blood sugar levels and may contribute to weight gain, which complicates diabetes management.

Processed Grain/Sugary Food	Reason to Avoid
White bread	High glycemic index, lacks fiber, rapidly increases blood sugar levels.
Regular pasta	Made from refined flour, which causes blood sugar spikes due to low fiber content.
White rice	High glycemic index, stripped of nutrients and fiber, quick impact on blood sugar.
Cereals with added sugar	High in sugar and often low in fiber, leading to rapid glucose increases.
Sugary breakfast bars	Often high in sugar and low in protein and fiber, leading to energy crashes.
Soda and sweetened	Very high in sugar, provides no nutritional

Processed Grain/Sugary Food	**Reason to Avoid**
beverages	value and spikes blood sugar.
Cakes, cookies, and pastries	High in sugar and unhealthy fats, contributing to poor blood glucose control.
Ice cream	High in sugar and fat, which can lead to weight gain and higher blood sugar.
Candy	Pure sugar with no nutritional benefits, causes immediate blood sugar spikes.
Sweetened yogurt	Often contains high amounts of added sugars, negating the potential benefits of yogurt.
Instant noodles	High in simple carbohydrates and often contain sugar and unhealthy fats.
Microwavable popcorn	Often contains added sugars and artificial ingredients that can increase blood sugar.
Frozen dinners	Processed with high levels of sugars and fats, generally low in nutrients.
Potato chips	High glycemic index and typically very salty, contributing to poor health outcomes.
Pretzels	Made from refined flour, high in salt and quick to impact blood sugar.

Processed Grain/Sugary Food	Reason to Avoid
Cornflakes	Highly processed, low in fiber, and often high in added sugars.
Flavored coffees	High in syrups and sugars, contributing to significant sugar intake.
Energy drinks	High sugar content and other harmful additives that spike blood sugar.
Packaged cookies	Refined grains, high in sugar and fats, lacking beneficial nutrients.
Doughnuts	Deep-fried and sugar-laden, very poor for blood sugar and overall health.

Consuming these foods can lead to difficulties in managing diabetes and increase the risk of diabetes-related complications. It's best to replace them with healthier options, such as whole grains (like whole wheat bread and pasta, brown rice), natural sugars (found in fruits), and snacks rich in fiber and protein. These healthier choices help maintain stable blood sugar levels, provide essential nutrients, and support overall health.

High-Fat Foods

Managing type 2 diabetes effectively includes being mindful of high-fat foods that can negatively impact blood sugar control and overall health.

High-Fat Food	Reasons to Avoid
Butter	High in saturated fats, which can raise cholesterol levels and increase the risk of heart disease.
Lard	Predominantly saturated fats, contributing to poor cardiovascular health.
Cream	Contains high levels of saturated fat, which can lead to weight gain and increased insulin resistance.
Full-fat cheese	High in saturated fat and calories, potentially leading to obesity, a risk factor for diabetes.
Regular ice cream	Loaded with sugar and saturated fats, which can spike blood sugar levels and contribute to weight gain.
Fatty cuts of beef	High in saturated fats, increasing the risk of high cholesterol and heart disease.
Fatty cuts of pork	Similar to fatty beef, it's high in saturated fats and

High-Fat Food	Reasons to Avoid
	can affect heart health negatively.
Bacon	Contains both saturated fats and sodium, which can impact heart health and blood pressure.
Sausages	High in fats and often contain additives and high levels of sodium.
Fried chicken	The frying process adds excessive saturated fats and calories.
Potato chips	Typically high in trans and saturated fats due to deep-frying, leading to increased heart risks.
Pastries (cakes, pies)	Loaded with sugars and unhealthy fats, which can lead to blood sugar spikes and weight gain.
Margarine	Often contains trans fats, which are linked to increased heart disease risk and inflammation.
Commercially fried foods	High in trans fats and unhealthy saturated fats, worsening heart health.
Regular salad dressings	High in calories and saturated fats, especially cream-based varieties.
Mayonnaise	High in calories and fats, which can contribute to weight gain if consumed in large amounts.
Palm oil	High in saturated fats, potentially leading to higher cholesterol levels.

High-Fat Food	Reasons to Avoid
Coconut oil	Contains a high level of saturated fats, which can elevate cholesterol levels.
Store-bought smoothies	Often high in sugars and fats, misleadingly unhealthy due to their 'healthy' branding.
Pizza	High in saturated fat and calories, particularly with high-fat toppings like pepperoni and extra cheese.

Individuals with type 2 diabetes are advised to limit these foods as part of their dietary strategy to manage their condition. The high content of unhealthy fats in these foods can exacerbate insulin resistance, negatively affect lipid profiles, and increase the risk of cardiovascular disease, which is already a concern for those with diabetes. Opting for lower-fat alternatives and focusing on a diet rich in vegetables, fruits, lean proteins, and whole grains can support better blood sugar control and overall health.

Sodium-Rich Foods

In managing type 2 diabetes, it's important to pay attention not just to sugar and carbohydrate intake but also to sodium consumption. Excessive sodium can lead to high blood pressure, which increases the risk of heart disease — a common concern for those with diabetes.

Sodium-Rich Food	Reasons to Avoid
Canned soups	Often contain high levels of sodium used as a preservative, which can significantly increase blood pressure.
Processed meats	Such as sausages, hot dogs, and bacon are cured with salt, leading to high sodium content.
Pickles	Preserved with a large amount of sodium, which helps maintain crunchiness but raises sodium levels.
Salted nuts	Added salt increases sodium intake, which can contribute to hypertension.
Instant noodles	Contain high levels of sodium in seasonings, posing risks for blood pressure spikes.

Sodium-Rich Food	Reasons to Avoid
Frozen dinners	Often have high sodium content to enhance flavor and preserve the food longer.
Regular cheese	Contains natural sodium and additional salt during processing.
Salted butter	Higher sodium content compared to unsalted varieties, contributing to increased dietary sodium.
Soy sauce	Very high in sodium, making even small amounts a significant source.
Table salt	Directly increases sodium intake, significantly affecting blood pressure control.
Salad dressings	Store-bought versions are typically high in sodium to enhance flavor and shelf life.
Canned vegetables	Often preserved with salt, which can be avoided by rinsing them under water or choosing fresh alternatives.
Fast food	Items like burgers, fries, and others are generally high in sodium for flavor enhancement.

Sodium-Rich Food	Reasons to Avoid
Salted snacks	Such as chips, pretzels, and crackers are major contributors to excessive sodium intake.
Deli meats	High sodium content due to curing, seasoning, and preservation processes.
Bouillon cubes	Used to enhance flavor in cooking but contain a high level of sodium.
Seasoning salts	Such as garlic salt or onion salt, which are primarily composed of sodium chloride.
Marinated and pre-seasoned meats	Often contain high levels of sodium to enhance taste and preserve the product.
Sports drinks	Can contain high levels of added salts to replenish electrolytes, contributing to overall sodium consumption.
Barbecue sauce	Typically contains high amounts of sodium for flavoring.

It is advisable for individuals with type 2 diabetes to read food labels carefully and choose lower-sodium or no-salt-added versions of these foods when possible. Cooking at home and using fresh ingredients also allows better control over sodium intake, which can help manage blood pressure and reduce the risk of cardiovascular complications associated with diabetes.

Nutritional Tips for Eating Out

Making Smart Choices in Restaurants

Eating out can be a delightful experience, but for those managing type 2 diabetes, it poses unique challenges, particularly in maintaining a diet that's beneficial for blood sugar control. Making smart choices in restaurants involves more than just avoiding sugar; it requires a comprehensive approach to select meals that are nutritious, appropriately portioned, and low in unhealthy fats and sodium.

Start by reviewing the menu online ahead of your visit if possible. Many restaurants offer nutritional information, allowing you to plan your meal before you arrive. This preparation prevents rushed decisions and helps you stay within your dietary goals. Look for dishes that emphasize grilled, baked, steamed, or broiled options rather than fried or sautéed ones, as cooking methods can greatly influence the calorie and fat content of a meal.

Ask for dressings, sauces, and gravies to be served on the side. This small step not only helps you control the amount you consume, it also allows you to assess the ingredient quality and avoid unnecessary sugars or fats often found in these additions. Similarly, be cautious with condiments like ketchup or barbecue sauce, which can be packed with sugar and sodium.

Opt for dishes rich in vegetables and lean proteins. Fish, chicken, or plant-based protein sources like beans and lentils are excellent choices. These not only offer high-quality protein but also help slow down the absorption of glucose into your bloodstream, aiding in blood sugar stabilization. When it comes to carbohydrates, choose whole grains like brown rice or whole wheat pasta, if available, and always be mindful of portion sizes. A good rule of thumb is to have carbohydrates cover no more than a quarter of your plate.

If the portion sizes at the restaurant are large, consider asking for a half portion or a children's size if it's more in line with dietary recommendations. Alternatively, you can share a dish with someone else or ask for a to-go box at the start of the meal and set aside part of your dish to avoid overeating.

When it comes to beverages, stick to water, unsweetened tea, or black coffee. Sugary drinks, including sodas and alcohol, can rapidly increase blood sugar levels and provide no nutritional benefit. If you prefer a drink with flavor, consider a slice of lemon or lime to add to your water.

Lastly, don't hesitate to communicate with your server about your dietary needs. Most restaurants are willing to accommodate requests from guests who have specific health-related dietary restrictions. Asking for substitutions or special preparations can make a significant difference in how a meal fits into your diabetes management plan.

By implementing these strategies, dining out can still be an enjoyable and integral part of your social life without compromising your health goals. These mindful eating habits not only support diabetes management but also contribute to an overall healthier lifestyle.

Diabetes-Friendly Fast Food Options

Eating out, particularly at fast food restaurants, can be challenging for those managing type 2 diabetes, but it's not impossible. With careful choices, you can enjoy meals that fit within your dietary needs without compromising blood sugar control or overall health.

When choosing diabetes-friendly fast food options, focus on balance and portion control. Opt for items that combine lean proteins, healthy fats, and fibers while minimizing simple carbohydrates and sugars that can spike blood glucose levels. Start by selecting grilled over fried items, as grilled foods are typically lower in calories and fat.

Salads are often a good choice, but be cautious of high-calorie dressings, croutons, and additional toppings like bacon bits, which can quickly increase the fat and calorie content. Request dressings on the side to control the amount and choose vinaigrette over creamy dressings to keep it healthier.

Many fast food chains now offer wraps or sandwiches with whole grain or whole wheat options. Choose these over white bread products to increase your fiber intake, which helps slow the absorption of sugar. Be sure to skip or limit high-sugar sauces like ketchup or barbecue sauce, opting for mustard or low-fat mayonnaise instead.

Burger joints can also be part of a diabetes-friendly diet if approached carefully. Opt for a single patty and add extra vegetables like lettuce, tomatoes, and onions. Skip the cheese and high-calorie sauces, and if possible, choose a lettuce wrap instead of a bun to reduce carbohydrate intake.

For side dishes, bypass the fries and opt for side salads, fruit cups, or yogurt. These alternatives provide more nutrients and are generally lower in calories and fat. If a restaurant offers soup, choose broth-based soups instead of cream-based, and be aware of the sodium content.

When it comes to beverages, water is the best choice. Avoid sodas and sweetened beverages, which can cause a quick rise in blood sugar levels. If you desire something with flavor, consider unsweetened iced tea or coffee, and control the amount of any added sweetener or cream.

Chicken places often have grilled chicken options, such as grilled chicken pieces or salads with grilled chicken. Avoid anything battered or fried and check if the marinades or seasonings are high in sugar or sodium.

Mexican fast food can be a good option if you select dishes made with whole beans, brown rice, and plenty of vegetables. Avoid dishes with large amounts of cheese and sour cream. Consider taco salads (without the fried bowl) or burrito bowls, where you can control the ingredients like skipping rice and choosing more vegetables and lean proteins.

For breakfast options, many fast food outlets offer egg-based dishes. Choose options like an egg and cheese sandwich on whole grain, and skip high-carb items like pancakes and sweetened oatmeal. Be cautious of breakfast meats like sausage and bacon, which are high in saturated fats and sodium.

Always remember that preparation can make a big difference when eating out. Many restaurants offer nutritional information online, allowing you to plan what you'll order in advance. By knowing what to choose before you walk in or drive through, you can make smarter choices that will keep you on track with your diabetes management.

Supplements and Diabetes

Vitamins and Minerals in Diabetes Care

Managing type 2 diabetes involves more than just monitoring carbohydrate intake; it also requires a balanced intake of vitamins and minerals to support overall health and regulate blood sugar levels. Certain vitamins and minerals are particularly important for individuals dealing with diabetes, as they can influence glucose metabolism and insulin sensitivity.

Magnesium plays a critical role in the regulation of insulin action and glucose metabolism. Research suggests that higher dietary magnesium intake is associated with lower fasting glucose and insulin levels, which can help prevent complications associated with diabetes. Foods rich in magnesium include leafy greens, nuts, seeds, and whole grains.

Chromium is another essential mineral for carbohydrate and lipid metabolism. It enhances the action of insulin and is important in maintaining normal blood sugar levels. Whole grains, nuts, green beans, and broccoli are good sources of chromium, but some people with diabetes might benefit from chromium supplementation as part of their dietary management plan.

Vitamin D deficiency is commonly found in individuals with type 2 diabetes. Adequate levels of vitamin D support insulin secretion and sensitivity, which are crucial for glucose regulation. Safe sun exposure, fatty fish, fortified dairy products, and vitamin D supplements can help maintain optimal levels.

Antioxidant vitamins such as Vitamin E and Vitamin C are also vital. Vitamin E helps combat oxidative stress, which is elevated in diabetes and can lead to complications. Vitamin C helps in the regeneration of vitamin E and improves endothelial function, reducing the risk of cardiovascular diseases. Sources include nuts, seeds, citrus fruits, and green vegetables.

B vitamins, especially Vitamin B1 (thiamine), B6, and B12, are important for nerve health and the prevention of diabetic neuropathy, a common complication of diabetes. Meat, fish, eggs, and dairy products are good sources of B vitamins. For those who struggle to get enough from their diet, supplements might be necessary.

Zinc is another mineral that helps with glucose control by enhancing insulin action and is involved in the processing, storage, and secretion of insulin. Meat, shellfish, legumes, and seeds are excellent sources of zinc.

Calcium and potassium are important for overall health and maintaining optimal blood pressure, which can be problematic in diabetes management. Low-fat dairy products, leafy greens, and bananas are recommended to ensure sufficient calcium and potassium intake.

It's essential for those managing type 2 diabetes to discuss with healthcare providers before starting any supplements, as some might interfere with medications or have side effects. A well-planned diet, possibly supplemented with vitamins and minerals as necessary, is a cornerstone of effective diabetes management, helping to stabilize blood sugar and prevent the development of complications.

Herbal Supplements and Their Effects

Managing type 2 diabetes often involves monitoring diet and medications closely, but herbal supplements have also become popular for their potential to support blood sugar control and overall health. While these supplements can complement diabetes management, it's crucial to approach them with careful consideration and preferably under the guidance of a healthcare provider.

Cinnamon is one of the most widely recognized herbal supplements linked to diabetes management. Studies suggest that it may improve blood sugar levels by increasing insulin sensitivity and slowing the breakdown of carbohydrates in the digestive tract. However, excessive consumption could potentially cause liver damage, emphasizing the need for moderation.

Bitter melon resembles a cucumber with a rough skin and is traditionally used in Asia, Africa, and South America to help lower blood sugar levels. Research indicates that it can act in a manner similar to insulin, helping glucose move into cells and thus lowering blood sugar levels. Yet, its long-term effects remain poorly understood, and it may interact with diabetes medications.

Fenugreek seeds contain fiber and other chemicals that may slow digestion and the body's absorption of carbohydrates and sugar. The seeds may also help improve how the body uses sugar and increase the amount of insulin released. Despite these benefits, fenugreek should be used cautiously as it can interact with blood thinning medications.

Ginseng, notably American and Korean varieties, has been observed to improve pancreatic cell function, boost insulin production, and enhance the uptake of blood sugar in tissues. Regular use of ginseng might help improve blood sugar control and glycaemic control. However, ginseng may also interact with other medications, including warfarin and those that affect blood sugar levels.

Alpha-lipoic acid, a naturally occurring fatty acid that can be found in foods like spinach, broccoli, and potatoes, is another supplement used for diabetes treatment. It has antioxidant properties that may help reduce oxidative stress and improve insulin sensitivity. However, it's known to cause potential side effects like nausea, rash, and can lower blood sugar levels significantly.

Chromium is a trace mineral believed to enhance the action of insulin. While it is involved in carbohydrate, fat, and protein metabolism, studies on its benefits for diabetes management are mixed, and high doses might cause kidney damage.

Berberine, a compound found in several plants, has shown promise in reducing blood sugar levels comparable to some diabetes drugs. It works by improving insulin sensitivity and increasing glycolysis, helping break down sugars inside cells. Berberine also affects various other bodily systems and can lead to digestive side effects.

It is essential for those considering herbal supplements to discuss them with their healthcare provider. Many supplements can interact with traditional medications and may not be suitable for everyone. Ensuring quality and verifying the purity of supplements is also critical, as the market is not as strictly regulated as prescription medications. This cautious approach will help mitigate any risks and align with overall diabetes management and health goals.

Monitoring and Adjusting Your Diet

Regular Blood Sugar Monitoring

Regular blood sugar monitoring is a cornerstone of effective diabetes management. It provides immediate feedback on how different foods and activities affect blood glucose levels, enabling individuals with type 2 diabetes to make informed decisions about their diet and lifestyle. By keeping track of blood sugar levels throughout the day, you can learn to anticipate how your body responds to certain foods and identify patterns that may require adjustments in your meal planning.

For most individuals managing type 2 diabetes, testing blood sugar is recommended at various times to get a complete picture of glucose control. Typically, this includes testing fasting blood glucose in the morning, before meals, two hours after meals, and at bedtime. This regimen can vary depending on individual health needs and the recommendations of a healthcare provider.

The process involves using a blood glucose meter, which requires a small blood sample usually taken from the fingertip. The blood is placed on a test strip inserted into the meter, which then reads and displays the glucose level. These meters vary in features, cost, and the size of the blood sample needed. Some newer models allow for testing at alternate sites, such as the forearm or palm, which may be less painful than fingertip testing.

Maintaining a logbook or using a digital app to record blood sugar readings along with notes on meals, activity, and medication is highly beneficial. This record keeping is invaluable for recognizing the effects of dietary choices on blood glucose levels. For example, if you notice that your blood sugar spikes after eating certain types of fruits or carbohydrate-rich foods, you might adjust your diet to include lower-glycemic options or alter your meal portions or timing.

Regular consultations with a healthcare provider are essential to interpret the results accurately and make necessary adjustments to your diabetes management plan. Your doctor or diabetes educator can help you set target blood sugar levels, understand your results, and decide if changes to your medication, diet, or exercise routines are needed based on your logs.

In addition to regular day-to-day monitoring, periodic A1C tests, which measure average blood glucose levels over the past two to three months, are used to assess long-term glucose control. An A1C level of 7% or lower is typically the goal for many adults with diabetes, but these targets can vary based on individual health profiles.

The ultimate goal of regular blood sugar monitoring is to maintain blood glucose levels within target ranges as much as possible, thereby reducing the risk of diabetes-related complications such as neuropathy, retinopathy, and cardiovascular disease. Adjusting your diet based on monitoring results can lead to significant improvements in glucose control and overall health. It allows for a proactive approach to managing type 2 diabetes, empowering individuals to take control of their condition and enhance their quality of life.

When to Adjust Your Diet

Adjusting your diet is a key component of managing type 2 diabetes effectively. Monitoring your blood sugar levels regularly gives you direct feedback on how your body reacts to different foods and meals. When you notice consistent patterns in blood sugar fluctuations that could be tied to specific foods or meals, it's time to consider making dietary adjustments. This feedback loop enables you to tailor your diet to better suit your body's needs, leading to more stable blood sugar levels.

If you experience hypoglycemic episodes, where your blood sugar drops too low, this could indicate that your carbohydrate intake is too low or that you're taking too much diabetes medication relative to the amount of food you consume. On the other hand, consistently high blood sugar levels after meals might suggest that you are consuming too many carbohydrates, or your medication needs adjustment.

Another indicator that you should adjust your diet is weight change. If you are losing weight without trying, it could mean your diet does not provide enough calories or carbohydrates. Alternatively, unintended weight gain might suggest that your diet is too calorie-dense, and adjustments may be necessary to help you achieve a healthier weight.

Consultation with healthcare professionals is vital whenever you make changes to your diet. A dietitian can help analyze your food diary and blood sugar logs to recommend dietary adjustments that align with your health goals. They can also ensure that you maintain nutritional balance, which is crucial for overall health, especially in managing a chronic condition like diabetes.

Regular visits to your healthcare provider are also important as they might need to adjust your diabetes medication based on changes in your diet, weight, and lifestyle. It's essential to have a collaborative approach with your healthcare team to ensure that all aspects of your health are considered.

The seasons and your activity levels can also dictate when to adjust your diet. For instance, you might be more active in the summer, requiring adjustments in carbohydrate intake or meal timing to prevent low blood sugar levels during or after exercise. Similarly, holiday seasons might require adjustments to handle different types of foods and possibly more eating out.

Finally, listen to your body. It can tell you a lot about how well your diet is working for you. Feelings of tiredness, lethargy, or lack of focus can be related to improper blood sugar control and might require dietary adjustments. Adjusting your diet is not a one-time task but an ongoing process that can help you lead a healthier life with type 2 diabetes.

Working with a Dietitian or Nutritionist

Working with a dietitian or nutritionist can be immensely beneficial for individuals managing type 2 diabetes. These professionals specialize in creating personalized nutrition plans tailored to your specific health needs, preferences, and lifestyle. Here's how collaborating with a dietitian or nutritionist can support you in effectively using the Type 2 Diabetes Food List:

1. **Personalized Guidance**: Dietitians and nutritionists assess your current diet, medical history, and individual health goals to create a customized nutrition plan that aligns with your needs. They take into account factors such as your blood sugar levels, weight, activity level, and any medications you may be taking to design a diet that optimizes your health outcomes.

2. **Education and Empowerment**: These professionals provide valuable education about nutrition, helping you understand how different foods affect your blood sugar levels and overall health. They can teach you how to read food labels, plan balanced meals, and make healthier food choices both at home and when dining out. By

empowering you with knowledge, they enable you to take control of your diet and effectively manage your diabetes.

3. **Support and Accountability**: Working with a dietitian or nutritionist offers ongoing support and accountability on your journey to better health. They can help you set realistic goals, track your progress, and provide motivation and encouragement along the way. Regular appointments allow you to discuss any challenges or concerns you may encounter and receive personalized guidance to overcome them.

4. **Nutrition Therapy**: For individuals with more complex medical conditions or specific dietary restrictions, dietitians and nutritionists can provide nutrition therapy. This involves using diet as a therapeutic intervention to manage and prevent chronic diseases like type 2 diabetes. They may recommend specific dietary modifications, meal timing strategies, or supplementation to optimize your health outcomes.

5. **Monitoring and Adjustments**: Dietitians and nutritionists help you monitor your progress and make necessary adjustments to your diet plan as needed. They can review your blood sugar levels, weight, and other health markers to assess how well your current nutrition plan is working and make recommendations for modifications

accordingly. This ongoing monitoring ensures that your diet remains effective in managing your diabetes and promoting overall well-being.

6. **Collaboration with Healthcare Team**: Dietitians and nutritionists often collaborate closely with other members of your healthcare team, such as your primary care physician, endocrinologist, or diabetes educator. This interdisciplinary approach ensures that all aspects of your diabetes management are coordinated and optimized for the best possible outcomes.

Working with a dietitian or nutritionist is a valuable investment in your health for individuals with type 2 diabetes. Their expertise, personalized guidance, and ongoing support can help you navigate the complexities of managing your diet and achieve better control of your blood sugar levels. By collaborating with these professionals, you can develop lifelong healthy eating habits that support your overall well-being and quality of life.

Conclusion

In conclusion, the "Type 2 Diabetes Food List" serves as a valuable resource for individuals looking to manage their diabetes effectively through dietary choices. By providing comprehensive information on the types of foods to include and avoid, along with practical meal planning tips and recipes, this guide empowers readers to take control of their health and improve their overall well-being.

Through the guidance offered in this book, individuals with type 2 diabetes can learn how to make informed decisions about their diet, ensuring that they consume foods that help regulate blood sugar levels and reduce the risk of complications associated with diabetes. By emphasizing whole grains, vegetables, fruits, lean proteins, and healthy fats while limiting processed foods, sugars, and sodium-rich items, readers can adopt a balanced and nutritious eating plan that supports their health goals.

Moreover, the "Type 2 Diabetes Food List" encourages a holistic approach to diabetes management, recognizing the importance of regular physical activity, blood sugar monitoring, and consultation with healthcare professionals. By incorporating these lifestyle factors alongside dietary changes, individuals can achieve better glycemic control, maintain a healthy weight, and reduce the need for medication.

Ultimately, the goal of the "Type 2 Diabetes Food List" is to empower individuals with the knowledge and tools they need to make sustainable and positive changes to their diet and lifestyle. By embracing a diet rich in nutrient-dense foods and avoiding those that can exacerbate diabetes symptoms, readers can experience improved energy levels, better blood sugar management, and a higher quality of life overall.

In closing, the "Type 2 Diabetes Food List" serves as a roadmap to better health for individuals living with type 2 diabetes. By following the recommendations outlined in this guide and making mindful choices about the foods they consume, readers can take control of their diabetes and enjoy a happier, healthier future.

www.ingramcontent.com/pod-product-compliance
Lightning Source LLC
Chambersburg PA
CBHW050822250726

48653CB00006B/2382